The Vibrant Keto Diet Lunch Recipes

Super Tasty Recipes To Burn Fat and Improve Your Health

Otis Fisher

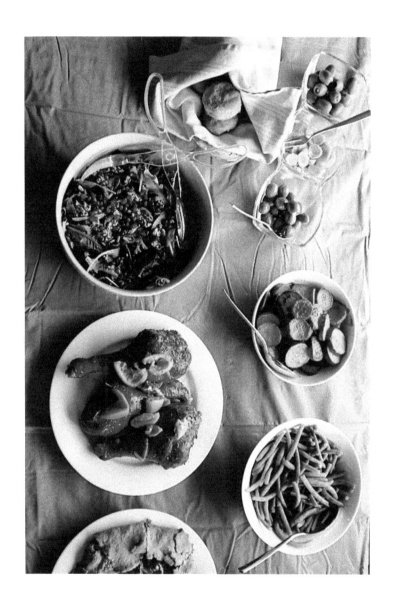

Table of contents

Scallion Mozzarella Cream Cheese Chaffle

Preparation Time: 1 hour 5 minutes

Cooking Time: 15 minutes

Servings: 4

Ingredients:

- 1 large egg
- 1/2 cup of shredded mozzarella
- 2 Tbsp. cream cheese
- 1 Tbsp. everything bagel seasoning
- 1-2 sliced scallions

Directions:

1. Turn on Chaffle maker to heat and oil it with Cooking spray. Beat egg in a small bowl.
2. Add in 1/2 cup mozzarella.
3. Whisk half of the mixture into the Chaffle maker and Cooking for 3-4 minutes. Remove chaffle and repeat with remaining mixture.
4. Let them cool, and then cover each chaffle with cream cheese, sprinkle with seasoning and scallions.

Nutrition:

Carbs 8 g

Fat 11 g

Protein 5 g

Calories 168

Lemony Fresh Herbs Chaffles

Preparation Time: 5 minutes

Cooking Time: 24 minutes

Servings: 6

Ingredients:

- 1/2 cup ground flaxseed
- 2 organic eggs
- 1/2 cup goat cheddar cheese, grated
- 2-4 tablespoons plain Greek yogurt
- 1 tablespoon avocado oil
- 1/2 teaspoon baking soda
- 1 teaspoon fresh lemon juice
- 2 tablespoons fresh chives, minced
- 1 tablespoon fresh basil, minced
- 1/2 tablespoon fresh mint, minced
- 1/4 tablespoon fresh thyme, minced
- 1/4 tablespoon fresh oregano, minced
- Salt and freshly ground black pepper

Directions:

1. Preheat a Chaffle iron and then grease it.
2. In a medium bowl, merge all ingredients and with a fork, mix until well combined.
3. Divide the mixture into 6 portions.

4. Place 1 portion of the mixture into preheated Chaffle iron and Cooking for about minutes or until golden brown.
5. Repeat with the remaining mixture.
6. Serve warm.

Nutrition:

Calories: 11

Fat: 7.9g

Carbohydrates: 3.7g

Sugar: 0.7g

Protein: 6.4g

Basil Chaffles

Preparation Time: 5 minutes

Cooking Time: 16 minutes

Servings: 3

Ingredients:

- 2 organic eggs, beaten
- 1/2 cup Mozzarella cheese, shredded
- 1 tablespoon Parmesan cheese, grated
- 1 teaspoon dried basil, crushed
- Pinch of salt

Directions:

1. Preheat a mini Chaffle iron and then grease it.
2. In a medium bowl, set all ingredients and mix until well combined.
3. Place 1/of the mixture into preheated Chaffle iron and Cooking for about 3-4 minutes or until golden brown.
4. Repeat with the remaining mixture.
5. Serve warm.

Nutrition:

Calories: 99

Fat: 4.2g

Carbohydrates: 0.4g

Sugar: 0.2g

Protein: 5.7g

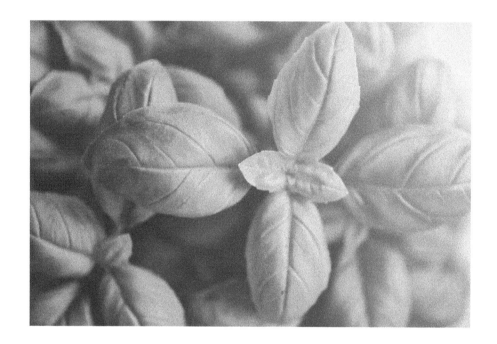

Scallion Cream Cheese Chaffle

Preparation Time: 5 minutes

Cooking Time: 20 minutes

Servings: 2

Ingredients:

- 1 large egg
- 1/2 cup of shredded mozzarella
- 2 Tbsp. cream cheese
- 1 Tbsp. everything bagel seasoning
- 1-2 sliced scallions

Directions:

1. Turn on Chaffle maker to heat and oil it with Cooking spray.
2. Beat egg in a small bowl.
3. Add in 1/2 cup mozzarella.
4. Whisk half of the mixture into the Chaffle maker and Cooking for 3-minutes.
5. Remove chaffle and repeat with remaining mixture.
6. Let them cool, and then cover each chaffle with cream cheese, sprinkle with seasoning and scallions.

Nutrition:

Carbs: 8 g

Fat: 11 g

Protein: 5 g

Calories: 168

Chicken Taco Chaffles

Preparation Time: 5 minutes

Cooking Time: 8 minutes

Servings: 2

Ingredients:

- 1/3 cup cooked grass-fed chicken, chopped
- 1 organic egg
- 1/3 cup Monterrey Jack cheese,
- 1/4 teaspoon taco seasoning

Directions:

1. Preheat a mini Chaffle iron and then grease it.
2. In a bowl, attach all the ingredients and mix until well combined.
3. Set half of the mixture into preheated Chaffle iron and Cooking for about 4 minutes or until golden brown.
4. Repeat with the remaining mixture.
5. Serve warm.

Nutrition:

Calories: 141

Fat: 8.9g

Carbohydrates: 1.1g

Sugar: 0.2g

Protein: 13.5g

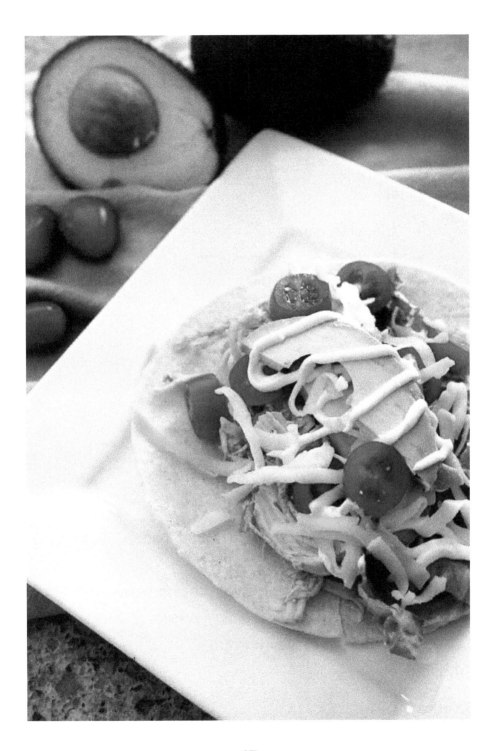

Crab Chaffles

Preparation Time: 5 minutes

Cooking Time: 25 minutes

Servings: 6

Ingredients:

- 1 lb. crab meat
- 1/3 cup Panko breadcrumbs
- 1 egg
- 2 tbsp. fat Greek yogurt
- 1 tsp. Dijon mustard
- 2 tbsp. parsley and chives, fresh
- 1 tsp. Italian seasoning
- 1 lemon, juiced

Directions:

1. Salt, pepper to taste
2. Add the meat. Mix well.
3. Form the mixture into round patties. Cooking 1 patty for 3 minutes.
4. Remove it and repeat the process with the remaining crab chaffle mixture. Once ready, remove and enjoy warm.

Nutrition:

Calories 99

Fats: 8 g

Carbs: 4 g

Protein: 16 g

Bacon and Egg Chaffles

Preparation Time: 5 minutes

Cooking Time: 10 minutes

Servings: 2

Ingredients:

- 2 eggs
- 4 tsp. collagen peptides, grass-fed
- 2 tbsp. pork panko
- 3 slices crispy bacon

Directions:

1. Warm up your mini Chaffle maker.
2. Combine the eggs, pork panko, and collagen peptides. Mix well. Divide the batter in two small bowls.
3. Once done, evenly distribute 1/2 of the crispy chopped bacon on the Chaffle maker.
4. Pour one bowl of the batter over the bacon. Cooking for 5 minutes and immediately repeat this step for the second chaffle.
5. Plate your cooked chaffles and sprinkle with extra Panko for an added crunch.
6. Enjoy!

Nutrition:

Calories: 266

Fats: 1g

Carbs: 11.2 g

Protein: 27 g

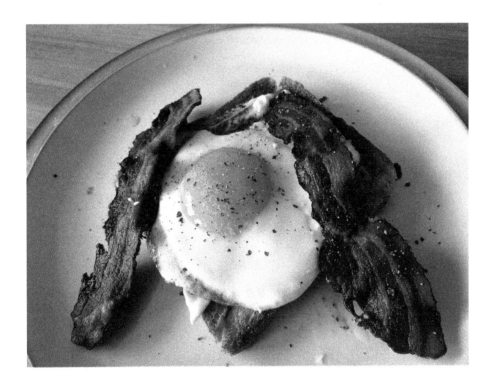

Chicken and Bacon Chaffles

Preparation Time: 5 minutes

Cooking Time: 8 minutes

Servings: 2

Ingredients:

- 1 organic egg, beaten
- 1/3 cup grass-fed cooked chicken, chopped
- 1 cooked bacon slice, crumbled
- 1/3 cup Pepper Jack cheese, shredded
- 1 teaspoon powdered ranch dressing

Directions:

1. Preheat a mini Chaffle iron and then grease it.
2. In a medium bowl, merge all ingredients and with a fork, mix until well blend.
3. Set half of the mixture into preheated Chaffle iron and Cooking for about 4 minutes or until golden brown.
4. Repeat with the remaining mixture.
5. Serve warm.

Nutrition:

Calories: 145

Fat: 9.4g

Carbohydrates: 1g

Sugar: 0.2g

Protein: 14.3g

Chaffle Katsu Sandwich

Preparation Time: 5 minutes

Cooking Time: 20 minutes

Servings: 4

Ingredients:

- For the chicken:
- 1/4 lb. boneless chicken thigh
- 1/8 tsp. salt
- 1/8 tsp. black pepper
- 1/2 cup almond flour
- 1 egg
- 3 oz. unflavored pork rinds
- 2 cup vegetable oil for deep frying For the brine:
- 2 cup of water
- 1 Tbsp. salt

For the sauce:

- 2 Tbsp. sugar-free ketchup
- 11/2 Tbsp. Worcestershire Sauce
- 1 Tbsp. oyster sauce
- 1 tsp. swerve/monk fruit For the chaffle:
- 2 egg
- 1 cup shredded mozzarella cheese

Directions:

1. Add brine ingredients in a large mixing bowl.
2. Add chicken and brine for 1 hour.
3. Pat chicken dry with a paper towel. Sprinkle with salt and pepper. Set aside.
4. Mix ketchup, oyster sauce, Worcestershire sauce, and swerve in a small mixing bowl.
5. Pulse pork rinds in a food processor, making fine crumbs.
6. Fill one bowl with flour, a second bowl with beaten eggs, and a third with crushed pork rinds.
7. Dip and coat each thigh in: flour, eggs, crushed pork rinds. Transfer on holding a plate.
8. Add oil to cover 1/2 inch of frying pan. Heat to 375F.
9. Once oil is hot, set heat to medium and add chicken. Cooking time depends on the chicken thickness.
10. Transfer to a drying rack.
11. Turn on Chaffle maker to heat and oil it with Cooking spray.
12. Beat egg in a small bowl.
13. Place 1/8 cup of cheese on Chaffle maker, then add1/4 of the egg mixture and top with 1/8 cup of cheese.
14. Cooking for 3-4 minutes.
15. Repeat for remaining batter.
16. Top chaffles with chicken katsu, 1 Tbsp. sauce, and another piece of chaffle.

Nutrition:

Carbs: 12 g

Fat: 1 g

Protein: 2 g

Calories: 57

Pork Rind Chaffles

Preparation Time: 5 minutes

Cooking Time: 10 minutes

Servings: 2

Ingredients:

- 1 organic egg, beaten
- 1/2 cup ground pork rinds
- 1/3 cup Mozzarella cheese, shredded
- Pinch of salt

Directions:

1. Preheat a mini Chaffle iron and then grease it.
2. In a bowl, set all the ingredients and beat until well blend.
3. Set half of the mixture into preheated Chaffle iron and Cooking for about 5 minutes or until golden brown.
4. Repeat with the remaining mixture.
5. Serve warm.

Nutrition:

Calories: 91

Fat: 5.9g

Carbohydrates: 0.3g

Sugar: 0.2g

Protein: 9.2g

Turkey Chaffles

Preparation Time: 5 minutes

Cooking Time: 16 minutes

Servings: 4

Ingredients:

- 1/2 cup cooked turkey meat, chopped
- 2 organic eggs, beaten
- 1/2 cup Parmesan cheese, grated
- 1/2 cup Mozzarella, shredded
- 1/4 teaspoon poultry seasoning
- 1/4 teaspoon onion powder

Directions:

1. Preheat a mini Chaffle iron and then grease it.
2. In a medium bowl, set all ingredients and mix until well combined.
3. Place 1/4 of the mixture into preheated Chaffle iron and Cooking for about 4 minutes or until golden brown.
4. Repeat with the remaining mixture.
5. Serve warm.

Nutrition:

Calories: 108

Fat: 1g

Carbohydrates: 0.5g

Sugar: 0.2g

Protein: 12.9g

Pepperoni Chaffles

Preparation Time: 5 minutes

Cooking Time: 5 minutes

Servings: 1

Ingredients:

- 1 organic egg, beaten
- 1/2 cup Mozzarella cheese, shredded
- 2 tablespoons turkey pepperoni slice, chopped
- 1 tablespoon sugar-free pizza sauce 1/4 teaspoon Italian seasoning

Directions:

1. Preheat a Chaffle iron and then grease it.
2. In a bowl, set all the ingredients and mix well.
3. Place the mixture into preheated Chaffle iron and Cooking for about 5 minutes or until golden brown.
4. Serve warm.

Nutrition:

Calories: 119

Fat: 7.g

Carbohydrates: 2.7g

Sugar: 0.9g

Protein: 10.3g

Hot Sauce Jalapeño Chaffles

Preparation Time: 5 minutes

Cooking Time: 8 minutes

Servings: 2

Ingredients:

- 1/2 cup plus 2 teaspoons Cheddar cheese, shredded and divided
- 1 organic egg, beaten
- 6 jalapeño pepper slices
- 1/4 teaspoon hot sauce
- Pinch of salt

Directions:

1. Preheat a mini Chaffle iron and then grease it.
2. In a bowl, place 1/2 cup of cheese and remaining ingredients and mix until well combined.
3. Place about 1 teaspoon of cheese in the bottom of the Chaffle maker for about seconds before adding the mixture.
4. Set half of the mixture into preheated Chaffle iron and Cooking for about 3-minutes or until golden brown.
5. Repeat with the remaining cheese and mixture.
6. Serve warm.

Nutrition:

Calories: 153

Fat: 12.2g

Carbohydrates: 0.7g

Sugar: 0.4g

Protein: 10.3g

Aioli Chicken Chaffle Sandwich

Preparation Time: 5 minutes

Cooking Time: 5 minutes

Servings: 1

Ingredients:

- 1/4 cup shredded rotisserie chicken
- 2 Tbsp. Kewpie mayo
- 1/2 tsp. lemon juice
- 1 grated garlic clove
- 1/4 green onion, chopped
- 1 egg
- 1/2 cup shredded mozzarella cheese

Directions:

1. Mix lemon juice and mayo in a small bowl.
2. Turn on Chaffle maker to heat and oil it with Cooking spray.
3. Beat egg in a small bowl.
4. Place 1/8 cup of cheese on Chaffle maker, then spread half of the egg mixture over it and top with 1/8 cup of cheese. Close and Cooking for 3-minutes.
5. Repeat for remaining batter.
6. Place chicken on chaffles and top with sauce. Sprinkle with chopped green onion.

Nutrition:

Carbs: 3 g

Fat: 42 g

Protein: 34 g

Calories: 545

Sage and Coconut Milk Chaffles

Preparation Time: 5 minutes

Cooking Time: 24 minutes

Servings: 6

Ingredients:

- 3/4 cup coconut flour, sifted
- 11/2 teaspoons organic baking powder
- 1/2 teaspoon dried ground sage
- 1/8 teaspoon garlic powder
- 1/8 teaspoon salt
- 1 organic egg
- 1 cup unsweetened coconut milk
- 1/4 cup water
- 11/2 tablespoons coconut oil, melted
- 1/2 cup cheddar cheese, shredded

Directions:

1. Preheat a Chaffle iron and then grease it.
2. In a bowl, add the flour, baking powder, sage, garlic powder and salt and mix well.
3. Add the egg, coconut milk, water and coconut oil and mix until a stiff mixture forms.
4. Add the cheese and gently stir to combine.
5. Divide the mixture into 6 portions.

6. Place 1 portion of the mixture into preheated Chaffle iron and Cooking for about 4 minutes or until golden brown.
7. Repeat with the remaining mixture.
8. Serve warm.

Nutrition:

Calories: 147

Net Carb: 2.2g

Fat: 13g

Saturated Fat: 10.7g

Carbohydrates: 2.

Sugar: 1.3g

Protein: 4g

Hot Ham Chaffles

Preparation Time: 5 minutes

Cooking Time: 4 minutes

Servings: 2

Ingredients:

- 1/2 cup mozzarella cheese, shredded
- 1 egg
- 1/4 cup ham, chopped
- 1/4 tsp. salt
- 2 tbsp. mayonnaise
- 1 tsp. Dijon mustard

Directions:

1. Preheat your Chaffle iron.
2. In the meantime, add the egg in a small mixing bowl and whisk.
3. Add in the ham, cheese, and salt. Mix to combine.
4. Scoop half the mixture using a spoon and pour into the hot Chaffle iron.
5. Close and Cooking for 4 minutes.
6. Remove the Chaffle and place on a large plate. Repeat the process with the remaining batter.
7. In a separate small bowl, attach the mayo and mustard. Mix together until smooth.

8. Slice the Chaffles in quarters and use the mayo mixture as the dip.

Nutrition:

Calories: 110

Fats: 12 g

Carbs: 6 g

Protein: 12 g

Egg and Seed Buns

Preparation Time: 10 minutes

Cooking Time: 50 minutes

Servings: 8

Ingredients

- 2 egg whites
- 1 cup sunflower seeds, ground
- 1/4 cup flax seeds, ground
- 5 Tbsp. psyllium husks
- 1 cup boiling hot water
- 2 tsp. baking powder
- Salt to taste

Directions

1. Combine all the dry ingredients.
2. Add the egg whites and blend until smooth.
3. Add boiling water and keep whisking.
4. Set line a baking sheet with parchment paper and drop the dough on it one spoonful at a time to form buns.
5. Bake at 356F for 50 minutes.
6. Serve.

Nutrition:

Calories: 91

Fat: 4.2g

Carb: 12.1g

Protein: 3.3g

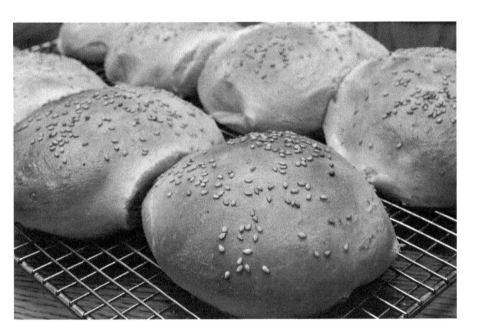

Garlic Bagels

Preparation Time: 10 minutes

Cooking Time: 15 minutes

Servings: 6

Ingredients

- 1/2 cup coconut flour
- 6 eggs
- 1 1/2 tsp. garlic powder
- 1/3 cup coconut oil
- 1/2 tsp. salt
- 1/2 tsp. baking powder

Directions

1. Preheat the oven to 400F.
2. Grease the bagel tin with coconut oil.
3. Whisk the eggs until it begins to form stiff peaks.
4. Combine the eggs, coconut oil, garlic powder, and salt in a bowl and whisk to combine.
5. Add the baking powder and the coconut flour and whisk to combine.
6. Pour the batter into the bagel tin and bake for 15 minutes.
7. Remove, cool, and serve.

Nutrition:

Calories: 193

Fat: 15g

Carb: 4.6g

Protein: 7.7g

Pumpkin Almond Cookies

Preparation Time: 10 minutes

Cooking Time: 30 minutes

Servings: 12

Ingredients

- 1 egg white
- 1 cup pumpkin puree
- 1 cup almond flour
- 1 cup almonds, ground
- 2 Tbsp. maple syrup, no sugar added
- 1/4 cup coconut flakes
- 1/4 cup lemon zest, grated

Directions

1. Combine flour, almonds, coconut flakes, and lemon zest.
2. Whisk the egg white until foamy and gradually add maple syrup.
3. Mix all ingredients together with pumpkin puree.
4. Set a baking sheet with parchment paper and add the cookies by the spoonful.
5. Bake at 300F for 30 minutes.
6. Serve.

Nutrition:

Calories: 315

Fat: 20g

Carb: 6g

Protein: 8.3g

Pumpkin Muffins

Preparation Time: 10 minutes

Cooking Time: 15 minutes

Servings: 8

Ingredients

- 1/2 cup butternut squash
- 1/2 cup low carb sweetener
- 4 eggs
- 1/4 tsp. baking soda
- 1/4 tsp. salt
- 1/2 tsp. ground nutmeg
- 1/2 tsp. ground cinnamon
- 1/2 tsp. ground cloves
- 1/2 tsp. ground ginger
- 1/4 cup plus 2 Tbsp. coconut flour

Directions

1. Preheat the oven to 350F.
2. Set a muffin pan by lining the muffin wells with liners. Grease the liners.
3. Place the puree, sweetener, and eggs in a bowl and blend well. Mix with a mixer.
4. Add the salt, flour, baking soda, nutmeg, cinnamon, cloves, and ginger to the wet ingredients and mix well. Let the batter sit and then mix again.

5. Set the muffin liners two-thirds full and bake for 15 minutes.
6. Cool and serve.

Nutrition:

Calories: 66

Fat: 3g

Carb: 6g

Protein: 4g

Buffalo hummus beef Chaffles

Preparation time: 15 minutes

Cooking time: 32 minutes

Servings: 4

Ingredients:

2 eggs

- 1 cup + 1/4 cup finely grated cheddar cheese, divided
- 2 chopped fresh scallions
- Salt and freshly ground black pepper
- 2 chicken breasts, cooked and diced
- 1/4 cup buffalo sauce
- 3 tbsp. low-carb hummus
- 2 celery stalks, chopped
- 1/4 cup crumbled blue cheese for topping

Directions:

1. Preheat the Chaffle iron.
2. In a medium bowl, mix the eggs, 1 cup of the cheddar cheese, scallions, salt, and black pepper,
3. Open the iron and add a quarter of the mixture. Close and Cooking until crispy, 7 minutes.
4. Transfer the chaffle to a plate and make 3 more chaffles in the same manner.

5. Set the oven to 400 f and set a baking sheet with parchment paper. Set aside.
6. Cut the chaffles into quarters and arrange them
7. on the baking sheet.
8. In a medium bowl, mix the chicken with the buffalo sauce, hummus, and celery.
9. Spoon the chicken mixture onto each quarter of chaffles and top with the remaining cheddar cheese.
10. Set the sheet in the oven and bake until the cheese melts, 4 minutes.
11. Remove from the oven and top with the blue cheese.
12. Servings afterward.

Nutrition:

Calories 552 Kcal

Fats 28.37g

Carbs 6.97g

Net carbs 6.07g

Protein 59.8g

Okonomiyaki chaffles

Preparation time: 20 minutes

Cooking time: 28 minutes

Servings: 4

Ingredients:

For the chaffles:

- 2 eggs, beaten
- 1 cup finely grated mozzarella cheese
- 1/2 tsp. baking powder
- 1/4 cup shredded radishes
- For the sauce:
- 2 tsp. coconut aminos
- 2 tbsp. sugar-free ketchup
- 1 tbsp. sugar-free maple syrup
- 2 tsp. Worcestershire sauce

For the topping:

- 1 tbsp. mayonnaise
- 2 tbsp. chopped fresh scallions
- 2 tbsp. bonito flakes
- 1 tsp. dried seaweed powder
- 1 tbsp. pickled ginger

Directions:

For the chaffles:

1. Preheat the Chaffle iron.
2. In a medium bowl, mix the eggs, mozzarella cheese, baking powder, and radishes.
3. Open the iron and add a quarter of the mixture. Close and Cooking until crispy, 7 minutes.
4. Transfer the chaffle to a plate and make a 3 more chaffles in the same manner.

For the sauce:

1. Combine the coconut aminos, ketchup, maple syrup, and Worcestershire sauce in a medium bowl and mix well.
2. For the topping:
3. In another mixing bowl, mix the mayonnaise, scallions, bonito flakes, seaweed powder, and ginger

To Servings:

1. Arrange the chaffles on four different plates and swirl the sauce on top. Spread the topping on the chaffles and Servings afterward.

Nutrition:

Calories 90 Kcal

Fats 3.32g

Carbs 2.97g

Net carbs 2.17g

Protein 12.09g

Keto Reuben chaffles

Preparation time: 15 minutes

Cooking time: 28 minutes

Servings: 4

Ingredients:

For the chaffles:

- 2 eggs, beaten
- 1 cup finely grated Swiss cheese
- 2 tsp. caraway seeds
- 1/8 tsp. salt
- 1/2 tsp. baking powder

For the sauce:

- 2 tbsp. sugar-free ketchup
- 3 tbsp. mayonnaise
- 1 tbsp. dill relish
- 1 tsp. hot sauce
- For the filling:
- 6 oz. pastrami
- 2 Swiss cheese slices
- 1/4 cup pickled radishes

Directions:

For the chaffles:

1. Preheat the Chaffle iron.

2. In a medium bowl, mix the eggs, Swiss cheese, caraway seeds, salt, and baking powder.
3. Open the iron and add a quarter of the mixture. Close and Cooking until crispy, 7 minutes.
4. Transfer the chaffle to a plate and make 3 more chaffles in the same manner.

For the sauce:

1. In another bowl, mix the ketchup, mayonnaise, dill relish, and hot sauce.

To assemble:

1. Divide on two chaffles; the sauce, the pastrami, swiss cheese slices, and pickled radishes.
2. Cover with the other chaffles; divide the sandwich in halves and Servings.

Nutrition:

Calories 316 Kcal

Fats 21.78g

Carbs 6.52g

Net carbs 5.42g

Protein 23.56g

Chicken Jalapeno Popper Chaffle

Preparation time: 5 minutes

Cooking time: 5 minutes

Servings: 2

Ingredients

- 1/2 cup canned chicken breast
- 1/4 cup cheddar cheese
- 1/8 cup parmesan cheese
- 1 egg
- 1 diced jalapeno (raw or pickled)
- 1/8 teaspoon onion powder
- 1/8 teaspoon of garlic powder
- 1 teaspoon of cream cheese

Directions:

1. Preheat mini Chaffle maker.
2. In an average bowl, add all ingredients and stir together till it's completely incorporated.
3. Half this mixture and Pour a part of the mixture into a mini Chaffle maker and Cooking for a minimum of five minutes.

Nutrition:

Calories 224 Kcal

Total Fat 21.8g

Cholesterol 134.6mg

Sodium 871mg

Total Carbohydrate 9.2g

Dietary Fiber 2.3g

Sugars 4.7g

Protein 18.5g

Jicama Hash Brown Chaffle

Preparation time: 5 minutes

Cooking time: 8 minutes

Servings: 2

Ingredients

- 1 large jicama root
- 1/2 onion chopped
- 2 garlic
- 2 eggs
- Salt and pepper

Directions:

Skin Jicama

1. Shred with food processor
2. Put the shredded jig in a large colander and sprinkle
3. 1-2 teaspoon salt, mix well and drain.
4. Squeeze out as much liquid as possible
5. 5-8 minutes microwave oven
6. Merge all the ingredients together
7. Whisk a little cheese on the Chaffle iron
8. Add 3T mixture and sprinkle a little more cheese
9. On the mixture
10. Set with a sunny side up egg!

Nutrition:

Calories 168 Kcal

Total Fat 11.8g

Cholesterol 121mg

Sodium 221.8mg

Total Carbohydrate 5.1g

Dietary Fiber 1.7g

Sugars 1.2g

Protein 10g20%

Chocolate Chip cooked Chaffle Cake

Preparation time: 10 minutes

Cooking time: 5 minutes

Servings: 2

Ingredients

Cake layer ingredients:

- 1 T butter melted
- 1 T Golden Monk Fruit Sweetener
- 1 egg yolk
- 1/8 tsp. vanilla essence
- 1/8 teaspoon cake batter extract
- 3 T almond flour
- 1/8 teaspoon baking powder
- 1 T Chocolate Chip Sugar-Free

Whipping cream frosting ingredients:

- 1 teaspoon unflavored gelatin
- 4 tsp. cold water
- 1 cup HWC
- 2 T sweetener

Directions:

1. Mix everything and Cooking on a mini Chaffle iron for 4 minutes. Repeat for each layer. I decided to make three.

2. Whipping cream frosting procedure

3. Set the beater and mixing bowl in the freezer for about 15 minutes to cool.

4. Sprinkle gelatin on cold water in a microwave-compatible bowl. Stir and "bloom". This takes about 5 minutes.

5. Microwave the gelatin mixture for 10 seconds. It becomes liquid. Stir to make sure everything is melted.

6. In a chilled mixing bowl, start whipping the cream at low speed. Add the confectionery sugar.

7. Move faster and observe that good peaks begin to form.

8. When the whipped cream has peaked, switch to low speed and squirt the melted liquid gelatin mixture slowly. Once in, switch to high speed and continue tapping until a hard peak is reached.

9. Set it in a piping bag and pipe the cake.

Nutrition:

Calories 84 Kcal

Total Fat 4.5g

Cholesterol 71.3mg

Sodium 122.3mg

Total Carbohydrate 5.3g

Dietary Fiber 0.9g

Sugars 2.1g

Protein 6.1g

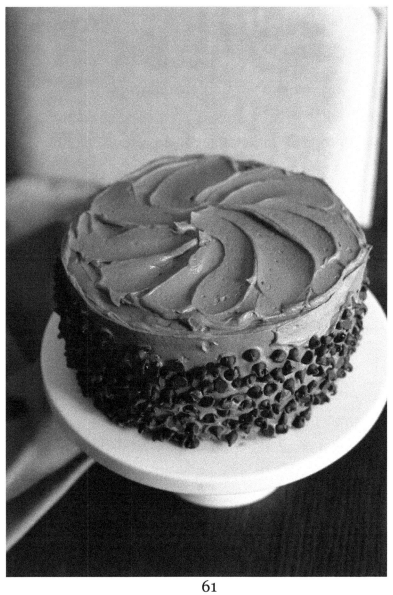

Keto Red Velvet Chaffle Cake

Preparation time: 10 minutes

Cooking time: 5 minutes

Servings: 2

Ingredients

- 2 Tbs. Dutch-processed cocoa
- 2 Tbs. Monk fruit Confectioner's
- 1 egg
- 2 drops of optional super drop food coloring
- 1/4 teaspoon baking powder
- 1 Tbs. Heavy Whipped Cream
- Frosted ingredients
- 2 Tbs. Monk fruit Confectioners
- 2 Tbs. cream cheese softens, room temperature
- 1/4 teaspoon transparent vanilla

Directions:

1. Put the eggs in a small bowl.
2. Attach the remaining ingredients and blend well until smooth and creamy.
3. Put half of the butter in a mini Chaffle pan and Cooking for 2 1/2 to 3 minutes until completely cooked.

4. Put the sweetener, cream cheese and vanilla in separate small pots. Mix the frosting until everything mixes well.
5. When the Chaffle cake has completely cooled to room temperature, spread the frosting.
6. Report makes two mini Chaffles

Nutrition:

Calories 75 Kcal

Total Fat 5.8g

Cholesterol 101.5mg

Sodium 39.8mg

Total Carbohydrate 4.1g

Dietary Fiber 2g

Sugars 0.4g

Protein 4.4g

Crunchy Fish and Chaffle Bites

Preparation Time: 10 minutes

Cooking Time: 15 minutes

Servings: 2

Ingredients:

- 1 lb. cod fillets, sliced into 4 slices
- 1 tsp. sea salt
- 1 tsp. garlic powder
- 1 egg, whisked
- 1 cup almond flour
- 2 tbsp. avocado oil

Chaffle Ingredients:

- 2 eggs
- 1/2 cup cheddar cheese
- 2 tbsp. almond flour
- 1/2 tsp. Italian seasoning

Directions:

1. Mix together chaffle ingredients in a bowl and make 4 squares.
2. Put the chaffles in a preheated chaffle maker.
3. Mix together the salt, pepper, and garlic powder in a mixing bowl. Toss the cod cubes in this mixture and let sit for 10 minutes.

4. Then dip each cod slice into the egg mixture and then into the almond flour.
5. Heat oil in skillet and fish cubes for about 2-3 minutes, until cooked and browned.
6. Serve on chaffles and enjoy!

Nutrition:

Protein: 38

Fat: 59

Carbohydrates: 11

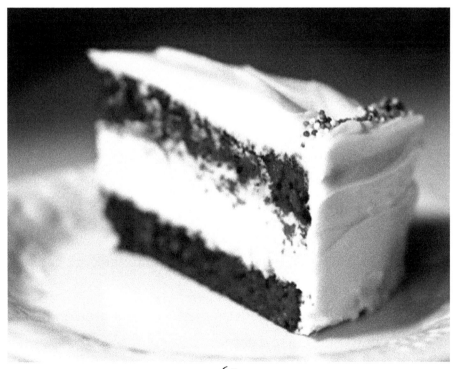

Grill Pork Chaffle Sandwich

Preparation Time: 10 minutes

Cooking Time: 15 minutes

Servings: 2

Ingredients:

- 1/2 cup mozzarella, shredded
- 1 egg
- I pinch garlic powder
- Pork Patty:
- 1/2 cup pork, minutes
- 1 tbsp. green onion, diced
- 1/2 tsp. Italian seasoning
- Lettuce leaves

Directions:

1. Preheat the square Chaffle maker and grease it.
2. Mix together egg, cheese and garlic powder in a small mixing bowl.
3. Pour batter in a preheated Chaffle maker and close the lid.
4. Make 2 chaffles from this batter.
5. Cooking chaffles for about 2-3 minutes until cooked through.
6. Meanwhile, mix together pork patty ingredients in a bowl and make 1 large patty.

7. Grill pork patty in a preheated grill for about 3-4 minutes per side until cooked through.
8. Arrange pork patty between two chaffles with lettuce leaves. Cut sandwich to make a triangular sandwich.
9. Enjoy!

Nutrition:

Protein: 48

Fat: 48

Carbohydrates: 4

Chaffle and Chicken Lunch Plate

Preparation Time: 10 minutes

Cooking Time: 15 minutes

Servings: 2

Ingredients:

- 1 large egg
- 1/2 cup jack cheese, shredded
- 1 pinch salt

For Serving:

- 1 chicken leg
- Salt
- Pepper
- 1 tsp. garlic
- 1 egg
- 1 tsp. avocado oil

Directions:

1. Heat your square Chaffle maker and grease with Cooking spray.
2. Pour Chaffle batter into the skillet and Cooking for about 3 minutes.
3. Meanwhile, heat oil in a pan, over medium heat.

4. Once the oil is hot, add chicken thigh and garlic then, Cooking for about 5 minutes. Flip and Cooking for another 3-4 minutes.
5. Season with salt and pepper and give them a good mix.
6. Transfer cooked thigh to plate.
7. Set the egg in the same pan for about 1-2 minutes according to your choice.
8. Once chaffles are cooked, serve with fried egg and chicken thigh.
9. Enjoy!

Nutrition:

Protein: 31

Fat: 66

Carbohydrates: 2

Chaffle Minutes Sandwich

Preparation Time: 10 minutes

Cooking Time: 10 minutes

Servings: 2

Ingredients:

- 1 large egg
- 1/8 cup almond flour
- 1/2 tsp. garlic powder
- 3/4 tsp. baking powder
- 1/2 cup shredded cheese

Sandwich Filling:

- 2 slices deli ham
- 2 slices tomatoes
- 1 slice cheddar cheese

Directions:

1. Grease your square Chaffle maker and preheat it on medium heat.
2. Mix together chaffle ingredients in a mixing bowl until well combined.
3. Pour batter into a square Chaffle and make two chaffles.
4. Once chaffles are cooked, remove from the maker.

5. For a sandwich, arrange deli ham, tomato slice and cheddar cheese between two chaffles.
6. Cut sandwich from the center.
7. Serve and enjoy!

Nutrition:

Protein: 29

Fat: 66

Carbohydrates: 4

Chicken Zinger Chaffle

Preparation Time: 10 minutes

Cooking Time: 15 minutes

Servings: 2

Ingredients:

- 1 chicken breast, cut into 2 pieces
- 1/2 cup coconut flour
- 1/4 cup finely grated Parmesan
- 1 tsp. paprika
- 1/2 tsp. garlic powder
- 1/2 tsp. onion powder
- 1 tsp. salt and pepper
- 1 egg beaten
- Avocado oil for frying
- Lettuce leaves
- BBQ sauce

Chaffle Ingredients:

- 4 oz. cheese
- 2 whole eggs
- 2 oz. almond flour
- 1/4 cup almond flour
- 1 tsp. baking powder

Directions:

1. Mix together chaffle ingredients in a bowl.
2. Pour the chaffle batter in preheated greased square chaffle maker.
3. Cooking chaffles for about 2 minutes until cooked through.
4. Make square chaffles from this batter.
5. Meanwhile mix together coconut flour, parmesan, paprika, garlic powder, onion powder salt and pepper in a bowl.
6. Dip chicken first in coconut flour mixture then in beaten egg.
7. Heat avocado oil in a skillet and Cooking chicken from both sides, until lightly brown and cooked.
8. Set chicken zinger between two chaffles with lettuce and BBQ sauce.
9. Enjoy!

Nutrition:

Protein: 30

Fat: 60

Carbohydrates: 9

Double Chicken Chaffles

Preparation Time: 10 minutes

Cooking Time: 5 minutes

Servings: 2

Ingredients:

- 1/2 cup boil shredded chicken
- 1/4 cup cheddar cheese
- 1/8 cup parmesan cheese
- 1 egg
- 1 tsp. Italian seasoning
- 1/8 tsp. garlic powder
- 1 tsp. cream cheese

Directions:

1. Preheat the Belgian Chaffle maker.
2. Mix together in chaffle ingredients in a bowl and mix together.
3. Sprinkle 1 tbsp. of cheese in a Chaffle maker and pour in chaffle batter.
4. Pour 1 tbsp. of cheese over batter and close the lid.
5. Cooking chaffles for about 4 to minutes.
6. Serve with a chicken zinger and enjoy the double chicken flavor.

Nutrition:

Protein: 30

Fat: 65

Carbohydrates: 5

Chaffles with Zucchini Topping

Preparation Time: 10 minutes

Cooking Time: 10 minutes

Servings: 2

Ingredients:

- 1 large egg
- 1 tbsp. almond flour
- 1 tbsp. full-fat Greek yogurt
- 1/8 tsp. baking powder
- 1/4 cup shredded Swiss cheese

Topping:

- 4oz. grill prawns
- 4 oz. steamed cauliflower mash
- 1/2 zucchini sliced
- 3 lettuce leaves
- 1 tomato, sliced
- 1 tbsp. flax seeds

Directions:

1. Make 3 chaffles with the given chaffles ingredients.
2. For serving, arrange lettuce leaves on each chaffle.
3. Top with zucchini slice, grill prawns, cauliflower mash and a tomato slice.
4. Drizzle flax seeds on top.

5. Serve and enjoy!

Nutrition:

Protein: 45

Fat: 47

Carbohydrates: 8

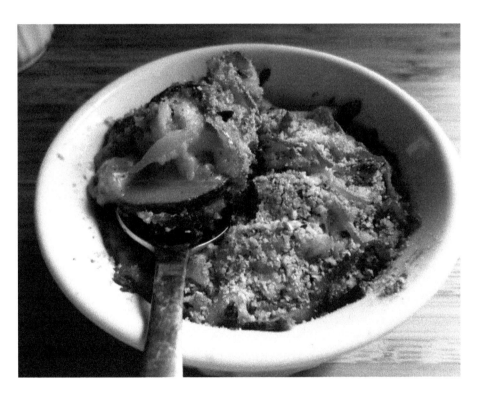

Chaffle with Melted Cheese and Bacon

Preparation Time: 10 minutes

Cooking Time: 15 minutes

Servings: 2

Ingredients:

- 1 egg
- 1/2 cup cheddar cheese, shredded
- 1 tbsp. parmesan cheese
- 3/4 tsp. coconut flour
- 1/4 tsp. baking powder
- 1/8 tsp. Italian Seasoning
- Pinch of salt
- 1/4 tsp. garlic powder

For Topping:

- 1 bacon sliced, Cooked and chopped
- 1/2 cup mozzarella cheese, shredded
- 1/4 tsp. parsley, chopped

Directions:

1. Preheat oven to 400 degrees.
2. Switch on your Mini Chaffle Maker and grease with Cooking spray.
3. Mix together chaffle ingredients in a mixing bowl until combined.

4. Spoon half of the batter in the center of the Chaffle maker and close the lid. Cooking chaffles for about 3 minutes until cooked.
5. Carefully remove chaffles from the maker.
6. Arrange chaffles in a greased baking tray.
7. Top with mozzarella cheese, chopped bacon and parsley.
8. And bake in the oven for 4-5 minutes.
9. Once the cheese is melted, remove from the oven.
10. Serve and enjoy!

Nutrition:

Protein: 28

Fat: 69

Carbohydrates: 3

Grilled Beefsteak and Chaffle

Preparation Time: 10 minutes

Cooking Time: 10 minutes

Servings: 1

Ingredients:

- 1 beefsteak rib eye
- 1 tsp. salt
- 1 tsp. pepper
- 1 tbsp. lime juice
- 1 tsp. garlic

Directions:

1. Prepare your grill for direct heat.
2. Mix together all spices and rub over beefsteak evenly.
3. Set the beef on the grill rack over medium heat.
4. Cover and Cooking steak for about6 to 8 minutes. Flip and Cooking for another 5 minutes until cooked through.
5. Serve with keto simple chaffle and enjoy!

Nutrition:

Protein: 51

Fat: 45

Carbohydrates: 4

Breakfast Cauliflower Chaffles and Tomatoes

Preparation Time: 10 minutes

Cooking Time: 15 minutes

Servings: 2

Ingredients:

- 1/2 cup cauliflower
- 1/4 tsp. garlic powder
- 1/4 tsp. black pepper
- 1/4 tsp. Salt
- 1/2 cup shredded cheddar cheese
- 1 egg

For Topping:

- 1 lettuce leave
- 1 tomato sliced
- 4 oz. cauliflower steamed, mashed
- 1 tsp. sesame seeds

Directions:

1. Add all chaffle ingredients into a blender and mix well.
2. Sprinkle 1/8 shredded cheese on the Chaffle maker and pour cauliflower mixture in a preheated Chaffle maker and sprinkle the rest of the cheese over it.

3. Cooking chaffles for about 4-5 minutes until cooked.
4. For serving, lay lettuce leaves over chaffle top with steamed cauliflower and tomato.
5. Drizzle sesame seeds on top.
6. Enjoy!

Nutrition:

Protein: 25

Fat: 65

Carbohydrates: 10

Classic Beef Chaffle

Preparation Time: 10 minutes

Cooking Time: 10 minutes

Servings: 2

Ingredients:

Batter:

- 1/2 pound ground beef
- 4 eggs
- 4-ounce cream cheese
- 1 cup grated mozzarella cheese
- Salt and pepper to taste
- 1 clove garlic, minced
- 1/2 teaspoon freshly chopped rosemary

Other:

- 2 tablespoons butter to brush the Chaffle maker
- 1/4 cup sour cream
- 2 tablespoons freshly chopped parsley for garnish

Directions:

1. Preheat the Chaffle maker.
2. Add the ground beef, eggs, cream cheese, grated mozzarella cheese, salt and pepper, minced garlic and freshly chopped rosemary to a bowl.

3. Brush the heated Chaffle maker with butter and add a few tablespoons of the batter.
4. Close the lid and Cooking for about 8-10 minutes depending on your Chaffle maker.
5. Serve each chaffle with a tablespoon of sour cream and freshly chopped parsley on top.
6. Serve and enjoy.

Nutrition:

Calories: 368

Fat: 24 g

Carbs: 2.1 g

Sugar: 0.4 g

Protein: 27.4 g

Sodium: 291 mg

Beef and Tomato Chaffle

Preparation Time: 10 minutes

Cooking Time: 15 minutes

Servings: 2

Ingredients:

Batter:

- 4 eggs
- 1/4 cup cream cheese
- 1 cup grated mozzarella cheese
- Salt and pepper to taste
- 1/4 cup almond flour
- 1 teaspoon freshly chopped dill
- Beef
- 1-pound beef loin
- Salt and pepper to taste
- 1 tablespoon balsamic vinegar
- 2 tablespoons olive oil
- 1 teaspoon freshly chopped rosemary

Other:

- 2 tablespoons Cooking spray to brush the Chaffle maker
- 4 tomato slices, for serving

Directions:

1. Preheat the Chaffle maker.
2. Add the eggs, cream cheese, grated mozzarella cheese, salt and pepper, almond flour and freshly chopped dill to a bowl.
3. Mix until combined and batter forms.
4. Brush the heated Chaffle maker with Cooking spray and add a few tablespoons of the batter.
5. Close the lid and Cooking for about 8-10 minutes depending on your Chaffle maker.
6. Meanwhile, heat the olive oil in a non-stick frying pan and season the beef loin with salt and pepper and freshly chopped rosemary.
7. Cooking the beef on each side for about 5 minutes and drizzle with some balsamic vinegar.
8. Serve each chaffle with a slice of tomato and cooked beef loin slices.

Nutrition:

Calories: 4

Fat: 35.8 g

Carbs: 3.3 g

Sugar: 0.8 g

Protein: 40.3 g

Sodium: 200 mg

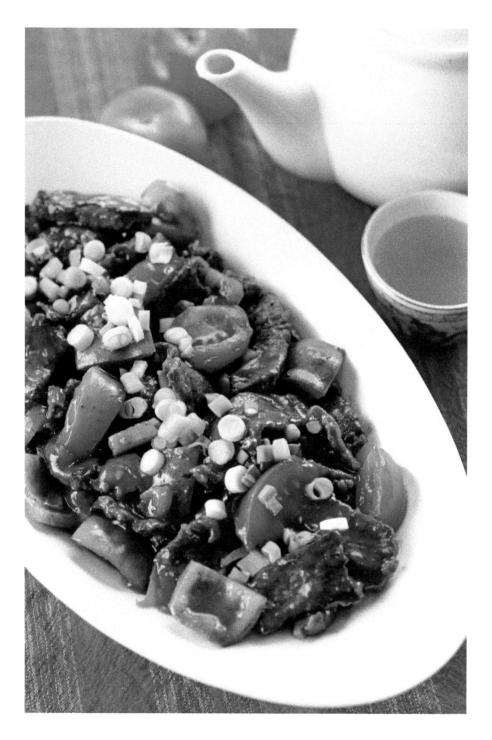

Classic Ground Pork Chaffle

Preparation Time: 10 minutes

Cooking Time: 15 minutes

Servings: 2

Ingredients:

- 1/2 pound ground pork
- 3 eggs
- 1/2 cup grated mozzarella cheese
- Salt and pepper to taste
- 1 clove garlic, minced
- 1 teaspoon dried oregano

Other:

- 2 tablespoons butter to brush the Chaffle maker
- 2 tablespoons freshly chopped parsley for garnish

Directions:

1. Preheat the Chaffle maker.
2. Add the ground pork, eggs, mozzarella cheese, salt and pepper, minced garlic and dried oregano to a bowl.
3. Mix until combined.
4. Brush the heated Chaffle maker with butter and add a few tablespoons of the batter.

5. Close the lid and Cooking for about 7-8 minutes depending on your Chaffle maker.
6. Serve with freshly chopped parsley.

Nutrition:

Calories: 192

Fat: 11.g

Carbs: 1 g

Sugar: 0.3 g

Protein: 20.2 g

Sodium: 142 mg

Keto Smore's

Preparation time: 5 minutes

Cooking time: 8 minutes

Servings: 2

Ingredients

- 1 large egg
- 1/2c. Mozzarella shredded
- 1/2 teaspoon of vanilla essence
- 2 tbs. swerve brown
- 1/2tbs plantain shell powder
- 1/4 teaspoon baking powder
- Pinch of pink salt
- 2 tbs. keto marshmallow cream fluff recipe

Directions:

1. Make a batch of keto marshmallow cream fluff.
2. Whisk the eggs until creamy.
3. Add vanilla and swerve brown and mix well.
4. Mix the shredded cheese and mix.
5. Next, add psyllium husk powder, baking powder and salt.
6. Mix until well mixed and let the dough rest for 3-4 minutes
7. Prepare / connect Chaffle maker to preheat.

8. Spread 1/2 batter to the Chaffle maker and Cooking for 3-4 minutes
9. Remove and install the cooling rack.
10. Cooking the other half of the dough in the same way, remove and let cool.
11. Once cool, assemble the chaffle with marshmallow fluff and chocolate.
12. Use 2 tablespoons marshmallow and 1/4 bar release chocolate.
13. Eat as it is or toast the melted and sticky small sandwich!

Nutrition:

Calories 120 Kcal

Total Fat 8.1g

Cholesterol 111.2mg

Sodium 1352.5mg

Total Carbohydrate 3.1g

Dietary Fiber 0.2g

Sugars 0.7g

Protein 8.3g

Cap'n Crunch Cereal Chaffle Cake

Preparation time: 5 minutes

Cooking time: 5 minutes

Servings: 2

Ingredients

- 1 egg
- 2 tablespoons almond flour
- 1/2 teaspoon coconut flour
- 1 tablespoon butter
- 1 tablespoon cream cheese
- Captain cereal flavor 20 drop
- 1/4 teaspoon vanilla essence
- 1/4 teaspoon baking powder
- 1 tablespoon confectionery
- 1/8 teaspoon xanthan gum

Directions:

1. Preheat mini Chaffle maker.
2. Merge all ingredients until smooth and creamy. Let the dough rest, until the flour has absorbed the liquid.
3. Add 2-3 tablespoons of batter to the Chaffle maker and Cooking for about 2 1/2 minutes.
4. Topped with fresh whipped cream (10 drops of captain cereal flavor and syrup!)

Nutrition:

Calories 154 Kcal

Total Fat 11.2g

Cholesterol 113.3mg

Sodium 96.9mg

Total Carbohydrate 5.9g

Dietary Fiber 1.7g

Sugars 2.7g

Protein 4.6g

Fried Pickle Chaffle Sticks

Preparation time: 5 minutes

Cooking time: 5 minutes

Servings: 2

Ingredients

- 1 egg
- 1/4 cup pork punk
- 1/2 cup mozzarella cheese
- 1 tablespoon of pickle juice
- 6-8 thin pickled slices

Directions:

1. Mix.
2. Add a thin layer to the Chaffle iron.
3. Suction excess juice from pickles.
4. Add the pickle slices and then mix another thin layer.
5. Cooking for 4 minutes.

Nutrition:

Calories 465 Kcal

Total Fat 22.7g

Cholesterol 250.1mg

Sodium 1863.2mg

Total Carbohydrate 3.3g

Dietary Fiber 1.4g

Sugars 1.5g

Protein 59.2g

Spicy Jalapeno Popper Chaffles

Preparation Time: 10 minutes

Cooking Time: 10 minutes

Servings: 1

Ingredients:

For the Chaffles:

- 1 egg
- 1 oz. cream cheese, softened
- 1 cup cheddar cheese, shredded

For the Toppings:

- 2 tbsp. bacon bits
- 1/2 tbsp. jalapenos

Directions:

1. Turn on the Chaffle maker. Preheat for up to 5 minutes.
2. Mix the chaffle ingredients.
3. Pour the batter onto the Chaffle maker.
4. Cooking the batter for 3-4 minutes until it's brown and crispy.
5. Remove the chaffle and repeat steps until all remaining batter have been used up.
6. Sprinkle bacon bits and a few jalapeno slices as toppings.

Nutrition:

Calories: 231

Carbohydrate: 2g

Fat: 18g

Protein: 13g

Eggnog Chaffles

Preparation Time: 15 minutes

Cooking Time: 10 minutes

Servings: 1

Ingredients:

- 1 egg, separated
- 1 egg yolk
- 1/2 cup mozzarella cheese, shredded
- 1/2 tsp. spiced rum
- 1 tsp. vanilla extract
- 1/4 tsp. nutmeg, dried
- A dash of cinnamon
- 1 tsp. coconut flour

For the Icing:

- 2 tbsp. cream cheese
- 1 tbsp. powdered sweetener
- 2 tsp. rum or rum extract

Directions:

1. Preheat the mini Chaffle maker.
2. Mix egg yolk in a small bowl until smooth.
3. Add in the sweetener and mix until the powder is completely dissolved.

4. Add the coconut flour, cinnamon, and nutmeg. Mix well.
5. In another bowl, mix rum, egg white, and vanilla. Whisk until well combined.
6. Throw in the yolk mixture with the egg white mixture. You should be able to form a thin batter.
7. Add the mozzarella cheese and combine with the mixture.
8. Separate the batter into two batches. Put 1/2 of the batter into the Chaffle maker and let it Cooking for 6 minutes until its solid.
9. Repeat until you've used up the remaining batter.
10. In a separate bowl, mix all the icing ingredients.
11. Top the cooked chaffles with the icing or you can use this as a dip.

Nutrition:

Calories: 266

Carbohydrates: 2g

Fat: 23g

Protein: 13g

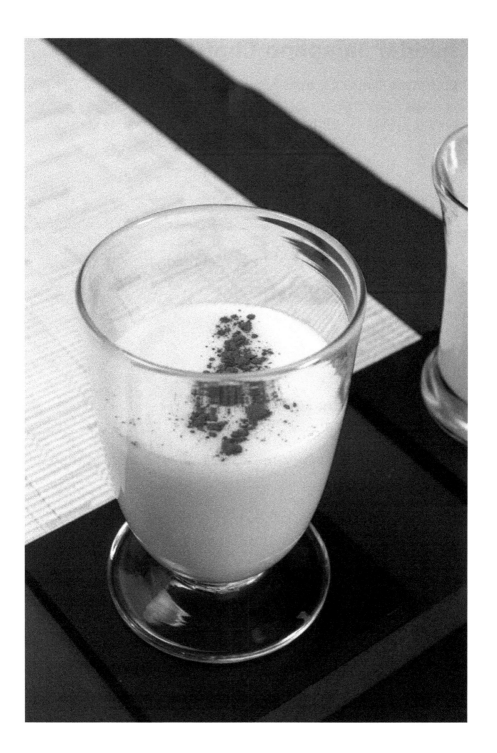

Cheddar Jalapeno Chaffles

Preparation Time: 15 minutes

Cooking Time: 10 minutes

Servings: 1

Ingredients:

- 1 egg
- 1/2 cup cheddar cheese, shredded
- 1 tbsp. almond flour
- 1 tbsp. jalapenos
- 1 tbsp. olive oil

Directions:

1. Preheat the Chaffle maker.
2. While waiting for the Chaffle maker to heat up, mix jalapeno, egg, cheese, and almond flour in a small mixing bowl.
3. Lightly grease the Chaffle maker with olive oil.
4. In the center of the Chaffle maker, carefully pour the chaffle batter. Spread the mixture evenly toward the edges.
5. Close the Chaffle maker lid and wait for 3-4 minutes for the mixture to Cooking. For an even crispier texture, wait for another 1-2 minutes.
6. Remove the chaffle. Let it cool before serving.

Nutrition:

Calories: 509

Carbohydrates: 5g

Fat: 45g

Protein: 23g

Low Carb Keto Broccoli Cheese Chaffles

Preparation Time: 5 minutes

Cooking Time: 5 minutes

Servings: 2

Ingredients:

- 1 cup broccoli, processed
- 1 cup shredded cheddar cheese
- 1/3 cup grated parmesan cheese
- 2 eggs, beats

Directions:

1. Spray the Cooking spray on the Chaffle iron and preheat.
2. Use a powerful blender or food processor to process the broccoli until rice consistency.
3. Mix all ingredients in a medium bowl.
4. Add 1/3 of the mixture to the Chaffle iron and Cooking for 4-5 minutes until golden.

Nutrition:

Calories: 160

Total Fat: 11.8g

Cholesterol: 121mg

Sodium: 221.8mg

Total Carbohydrate 5.1g

Sugars: 1.2g

Protein: 10g

Wonderful Chaffles

Preparation Time: 15 minutes

Cooking Time: 10 minutes

Servings: 1

Ingredients:

- 2 1/4 cups almond flour
- 1 teaspoon baking soda
- 1 teaspoon baking powder
- 1/2 teaspoon salt
- 1/4 cup butter
- 1/4 cup Swerve
- 1/2 cup mozzarella cheese, shredded
- 3 egg yolks
- 2 cups buttermilk
- 3 egg whites

Directions:

1. Preheat Chaffle iron. In a medium bowl, merge together almond flour, baking soda, baking powder and salt; set aside.
2. In a large bowl, merge cream butter and sweetener until light and fluffy. Attach mozzarella cheese and stir well.
3. Beat in egg yolks. Blend in flour mixture alternately with buttermilk.

4. In a mixing bowl, pour egg whites until stiff peaks form. Set 1/3 of the whites into the batter, and then quickly fold in remaining whites until no streaks remain.
5. Set Chaffle iron with non-stick Cooking spray, or lightly brush with oil. Ladle the batter onto preheated Chaffle iron. Cooking the chaffles until golden and crisp. Serve immediately.

Nutrition:

Calories 329,

Total Fat 11.1 g,

Cholesterol 126 mg,

Sodium 638 mg,

Total Carbohydrate 46.2 g,

Protein 10.8 g

Nutter Butter Chaffles

Preparation Time: 5 minutes

Cooking Time: 5 minutes

Servings: 2

Ingredients:

For the chaffles:

- 2 tbsp. sugar-free peanut butter powder
- 2 tbsp. maple (sugar-free) syrup
- 1 egg, beaten
- 1/4 cup finely grated mozzarella cheese
- 1/4 tsp. baking powder
- 1/4 tsp. almond butter
- 1/4 tsp. peanut butter extract
- 1 tbsp. softened cream cheese

For the frosting:

- 1/2 cup almond flour
- 1 cup peanut butter
- 3 tbsp. almond milk
- 1/2 tsp. vanilla extract
- 1/2 cup maple (sugar-free) syrup

Directions

1. Preheat the Chaffle iron.

2. Meanwhile, in a medium bowl, merge all the ingredients until smooth.
3. Open the iron and pour in half of the mixture.
4. Close the iron and Cooking until crispy, 6 to 7 minutes.
5. Remove the chaffle onto a plate and set aside.
6. Make a second chaffle with the remaining batter.
7. While the chaffles cool, make the frosting.
8. Pour the almond flour in a medium saucepan and stir-fry over medium heat until golden.
9. Transfer the almond flour to a blender and top with the remaining frosting ingredients. Process until smooth.
10. Spread the frosting on the chaffles and serve afterward.

Nutrition:

Calories 239,

Fats 19.48 g,

Net Carbs 7.92 g,

Protein 9.52 g

Buttery Rolls

Preparation Time: 5 minutes

Cooking Time: 25 minutes

Servings: 10

Ingredients

- 1/4 tsp. pink Himalayan salt
- 1/2 cup coconut flour
- 1/2 tsp. baking powder
- 3/4 cup water
- 2 Tbsp. psyllium husk powder
- 4 eggs
- 4 Tbsp. butter

Directions

1. In a bowl, combine the coconut flour, psyllium husk powder, salt, and baking powder.
2. Add the eggs into another bowl and beat together, then add in the water, melted butter, and mix well.
3. Combine the psyllium husk powder mixture with egg mixture. Mix until you get dough.
4. Mold the dough into 10 rolls then arrange on a parchment-lined baking sheet then place into a 350F preheated oven.
5. Bake for 30 to 35 minutes.
6. Cool and serve.

Nutrition:

Calories: 102

Fat: 7g

Carb: 5.8g

Protein: 3g